I0695933

Contents

Chapter 1: Introduction to Gastroparesis

Gastroparesis, a condition that affects the normal movement of the stomach muscles, can have a significant impact on a person's quality of life. In this chapter, we will dive deep into the world of gastroparesis, exploring its definition, causes, symptoms, diagnosis, treatment options, and most importantly, the role of diet in managing this condition.

1.1 What is Gastroparesis?

Imagine a well-orchestrated dance where the stomach muscles contract and relax in a coordinated manner to break down and propel food into the small intestine. Now, picture the disruption of this rhythm—a condition known as gastroparesis. Gastroparesis refers to delayed gastric emptying, where the stomach takes longer than usual to empty its contents into the small intestine.

Gastroparesis can occur due to various factors, including damage to the vagus nerve—a crucial nerve responsible for regulating stomach muscle movement. Diabetes, viral infections, certain medications, and autoimmune disorders are some common causes of gastroparesis.

1.2 Causes and Symptoms

Gastroparesis can stem from a range of underlying causes. One of the primary culprits is diabetes, which can damage the vagus nerve and impair stomach motility. Other causes include neurological conditions such as Parkinson's disease, multiple sclerosis, and stroke. Infections like Lyme disease or viral infections can also lead to gastroparesis.

The symptoms of gastroparesis can vary from person to person. Some common signs include nausea, vomiting, early satiety (feeling full after eating only small amounts of food), bloating, abdominal pain, and erratic blood sugar levels in individuals with diabetes.

1.3 Diagnosis and Treatment Options

Accurate diagnosis of gastroparesis is essential for effective management. The diagnostic process often involves a thorough medical history review, physical examination, and various tests. Gastric emptying studies, where a person ingests a meal or liquid containing a small amount of radioactive material, can provide valuable insights into the rate at which the stomach empties.

When it comes to treatment, a multimodal approach is typically employed to address the symptoms and underlying causes of gastroparesis. Medications that enhance stomach contractions (prokinetics), antiemetics to reduce nausea and vomiting, and pain medications may be prescribed. In severe cases, surgical interventions like gastric electrical stimulation or pyloroplasty may be considered.

1.4 Importance of Diet in Managing Gastroparesis

Diet plays a pivotal role in managing gastroparesis symptoms and improving the overall well-being of individuals living with this condition. While there is no one-size-fits-all diet for gastroparesis, making dietary modifications can significantly alleviate symptoms and enhance digestion.

The goals of a gastroparesis diet are to reduce the workload on the stomach, promote optimal digestion, prevent complications, and maintain proper nutrition. This entails consuming foods that are easier to digest, avoiding triggers that exacerbate symptoms, and adopting healthy eating habits.

Working closely with a healthcare team, including a registered dietitian or nutritionist, can be immensely beneficial. These professionals can provide personalized guidance on dietary modifications, portion control, and meal planning, ensuring that individuals with gastroparesis receive the necessary nutrients while managing their symptoms effectively.

In the following chapters, we will delve deeper into the specifics of the gastroparesis diet. We will explore the types of foods that are safe and well-tolerated, those that should be avoided or limited, and provide practical meal plans and recipes for gastroparesis-friendly meals. Additionally, we will discuss strategies for managing symptoms, special considerations for individuals with diabetes, and the importance of emotional well-being and support in navigating life with gastroparesis.

Gastroparesis may present challenges, but with the right knowledge, support, and dedication to a healthy lifestyle, individuals can regain control and improve their quality of life. Let us embark on this journey together, empowering ourselves with the tools and understanding necessary to manage gastroparesis and thrive despite its challenges.

Chapter 2: Understanding the Gastroparesis Diet

Welcome to Chapter 2 of our journey towards managing gastroparesis with a healthy diet. In this chapter, we will delve into the intricacies of the gastroparesis diet and explore how diet can impact gastroparesis symptoms. We will discuss the goals of a gastroparesis diet, the importance of working with a healthcare team, and the role of diet in managing this condition effectively.

2.1 How Diet Can Impact Gastroparesis Symptoms

The food we eat has a direct impact on our digestive system, and for individuals with gastroparesis, dietary choices can significantly influence their symptoms. Gastroparesis-friendly foods are typically those that are easy to digest, require less stomach muscle movement, and reduce the risk of complications such as delayed gastric emptying, bloating, and discomfort.

Understanding how different nutrients affect digestion is crucial for managing gastroparesis symptoms. For example, foods high in fat or fiber tend to take longer to digest and may exacerbate symptoms in some individuals. On the other hand, consuming smaller, frequent meals that are low in fat and fiber can help ease the workload on the stomach and promote better digestion.

2.2 Goals of a Gastroparesis Diet

The primary goals of a gastroparesis diet are to alleviate symptoms, maintain proper nutrition, and prevent complications. By making dietary modifications, individuals with gastroparesis can minimize discomfort, enhance digestion, and improve their overall well-being.

Some key goals of a gastroparesis diet include:

a) Reducing the workload on the stomach: Consuming smaller, more frequent meals allows the stomach to handle smaller volumes of food at a time, reducing the strain on the digestive system.

b) Promoting optimal digestion: Choosing foods that are easier to digest, such as cooked vegetables, lean proteins, and low-fiber grains, can help improve digestion and prevent symptoms like bloating and abdominal pain.

c) Preventing complications: Gastroparesis can increase the risk of blood sugar fluctuations, malnutrition, and bacterial overgrowth. A well-balanced diet that includes adequate nutrients, proper blood sugar management, and careful selection of food choices can help prevent these complications.

2.3 Working with a Healthcare Team

Managing gastroparesis effectively requires a multidisciplinary approach, and working closely with a healthcare team is essential. A team typically includes a gastroenterologist, registered dietitian or nutritionist, and possibly other specialists such as endocrinologists or neurologists, depending on the underlying cause of gastroparesis.

A registered dietitian or nutritionist plays a crucial role in guiding individuals with gastroparesis through dietary modifications. They can provide personalized recommendations, meal plans, and practical strategies to ensure individuals meet their nutritional needs while managing their symptoms effectively.

Collaborating with a healthcare team allows for comprehensive care, personalized advice, and ongoing support. Regular check-ins, adjustments to the treatment plan, and continuous education about managing gastroparesis can significantly improve outcomes and quality of life.

By working together with your healthcare team, you can gain valuable insights, tailor your diet to your specific needs, and receive the necessary support to navigate the challenges of living with gastroparesis.

In the next chapter, we will delve into the basics of a gastroparesis-friendly diet. We will explore dietary modifications, portion control guidelines, and provide tips for meal planning. Understanding these fundamentals will lay the foundation for building a gastroparesis diet that meets your individual needs and helps you manage your symptoms effectively.

Embrace the knowledge and support available to you, and let us continue on this journey towards better health and well-being despite the challenges of gastroparesis.

Chapter 3: The Basics of a Gastroparesis-Friendly Diet

Welcome to Chapter 3 of our comprehensive guide on managing gastroparesis with a healthy diet. In this chapter, we will delve into the fundamentals of a gastroparesis-friendly diet. We will explore the dietary modifications necessary for individuals with gastroparesis, guidelines for portion control, the importance of balancing nutritional needs, and practical tips for meal planning.

3.1 Dietary Modifications for Gastroparesis

Dietary modifications play a crucial role in managing gastroparesis symptoms and optimizing digestion. The key is to choose foods that are well-tolerated, easy to digest, and less likely to cause discomfort or delayed gastric emptying.

Here are some dietary modifications that can help individuals with gastroparesis:

a) Opt for smaller, more frequent meals: Consuming smaller meals throughout the day instead of three large meals can reduce the workload on the stomach and make digestion more manageable. Aim for 5-6 smaller meals spaced evenly throughout the day.

b) Choose soft, well-cooked foods: Foods that are soft, tender, and well-cooked are easier to digest. Consider incorporating options such as cooked vegetables, lean proteins like fish or poultry, and soft fruits like bananas or melons.

c) Avoid high-fat and high-fiber foods: Foods that are high in fat and fiber can be more challenging to digest and may exacerbate symptoms. Limit or avoid fried foods, fatty cuts of meat, whole grains, raw vegetables, and tough meats.

d) Be mindful of food texture: Foods with a smooth or pureed consistency are often better tolerated. Consider blending or pureeing foods to make them easier to digest. Soft foods like smoothies, soups, and pureed fruits or vegetables can be gentle on the stomach.

e) Stay hydrated: Adequate hydration is crucial for overall health and digestion. Sip water throughout the day and consider incorporating hydrating foods like clear broths, herbal teas, and fruits with high water content, such as watermelon or cucumbers.

Remember, dietary modifications may vary from person to person. It is essential to work closely with a registered dietitian or nutritionist who can provide personalized recommendations based on your specific needs and tolerances.

3.2 Guidelines for Portion Control

Portion control is vital for managing gastroparesis symptoms and promoting optimal digestion. Eating smaller portions allows the stomach to handle food more efficiently, reducing the risk of discomfort, bloating, and delayed gastric emptying.

Here are some guidelines for portion control:

a) Use smaller plates and bowls: Using smaller plates and bowls can create an illusion of a larger portion, helping you feel satisfied with less food. This can be particularly useful when consuming meals at home.

b) Focus on nutrient-dense foods: Choose foods that are rich in nutrients to ensure you receive the necessary nourishment even with smaller portions. Opt for lean proteins, nutrient-dense fruits and vegetables, and whole grains in appropriate quantities.

c) Listen to your body's signals: Pay attention to your body's hunger and fullness cues. Eat until you feel comfortably satisfied, rather than overeating or forcing yourself to finish a large portion.

d) Space out your meals: Allow sufficient time between meals to ensure your stomach has adequate time to digest the food. Aim for at least 2-3 hours between each meal or snack.

Remember, portion control is highly individualized. Work closely with your healthcare team to determine the portion sizes that best suit your needs and manage your symptoms effectively.

3.3 Balancing Nutritional Needs

Maintaining proper nutrition is crucial for individuals with gastroparesis. While dietary modifications may be necessary, it is essential to ensure that your diet includes all the necessary nutrients for optimal health and well-being.

Here are some tips for balancing nutritional needs:

a) Focus on nutrient-dense foods: Choose foods that provide a wide range of essential nutrients while being gentle on the stomach. Include lean proteins, such as chicken, fish, tofu, or legumes, as well as a variety of fruits, vegetables, whole grains, and healthy fats.

b) Consider supplements if needed: Gastroparesis can sometimes lead to nutritional deficiencies, particularly in vitamins and minerals. If necessary, work with your healthcare team to determine if you need any supplements to meet your nutritional needs.

c) Monitor blood sugar levels: For individuals with diabetes, managing blood sugar levels is crucial. Coordinate with your healthcare team to develop a meal plan that helps stabilize blood sugar levels while managing gastroparesis symptoms.

d) Experiment with different foods: Everyone's tolerance to different foods can vary. Keep a food diary and track how different foods make you feel. This can help you identify trigger foods and find a balance between optimal nutrition and symptom management.

3.4 Meal Planning Tips

Meal planning can be a helpful strategy for individuals with gastroparesis, as it allows for better control over food choices, portion sizes, and meal frequency. Here are some practical tips for meal planning with gastroparesis:

a) Plan meals and snacks in advance: Take time to plan your meals and snacks for the week. This can help ensure you have appropriate foods on hand and make it easier to adhere to your gastroparesis-friendly diet.

b) Cook in batches: Preparing larger quantities of gastroparesis-friendly meals and portioning them into smaller servings can save time and make it convenient to have ready-to-eat meals throughout the week.

c) Focus on variety: Aim to include a variety of foods from different food groups in your meal plan. This not only helps provide a wide range of nutrients but also makes mealtime more enjoyable.

d) Keep a stock of gentle-on-the-stomach foods: Keep a supply of easily digestible foods like low-fiber canned fruits, cooked vegetables, soft proteins, and easily digestible carbohydrates. This ensures you always have options available, even when you may not have the energy or ability to cook elaborate meals.

e) Be flexible and adapt: Gastroparesis symptoms can vary from day to day, so it's essential to be flexible with your meal plan. Listen to your body, make adjustments as needed, and don't be too hard on yourself if things don't go as planned.

By incorporating these meal planning tips into your routine, you can simplify the process of managing your gastroparesis diet while ensuring you meet your nutritional needs and minimize symptoms.

In the next chapter, we will explore in-depth the foods that are safe and well-tolerated in a gastroparesis diet. We will discuss high-fiber foods to include, lean proteins and plant-based options, healthy fats and oils, and ways to incorporate fruits and vegetables into your meals. Get ready to explore delicious and nourishing options that will support your journey towards managing gastroparesis effectively.

Remember, with careful planning and a positive mindset, you can create a gastroparesis-friendly diet that not only manages your symptoms but also allows you to enjoy a variety of delicious and nutritious foods.

Chapter 4: Foods to Include in Your Gastroparesis Diet

Welcome to Chapter 4 of our comprehensive guide on managing gastroparesis with a healthy diet. In this chapter, we will explore the foods that are safe and well-tolerated in a gastroparesis diet. We will discuss high-fiber foods for gastroparesis, lean proteins and plant-based options, healthy fats and oils, and ways to incorporate fruits and vegetables into your meals. Get ready to discover a variety of delicious and nourishing options that will support your journey towards managing gastroparesis effectively.

4.1 Introduction to Safe and Well-Tolerated Foods

When it comes to a gastroparesis diet, it is crucial to focus on foods that are safe and well-tolerated by individuals with delayed gastric emptying. These foods are typically easier to digest, require less stomach muscle movement, and reduce the risk of discomfort and delayed digestion.

Here are some safe and well-tolerated foods to include in your gastroparesis diet:

a) Cooked vegetables: Vegetables that are well-cooked and soft tend to be easier to digest. Consider options like mashed potatoes, pureed carrots, cooked zucchini, or squash.

b) Soft fruits: Opt for fruits that are gentle on the stomach, such as bananas, melons, and cooked apples. These fruits provide essential vitamins and minerals while being easier to digest compared to their raw counterparts.

c) Low-fiber grains: Choose grains that are low in fiber, such as white rice, white bread, or refined pasta. These options are generally more easily digested than whole grain alternatives.

d) Lean proteins: Include lean proteins in your diet to support muscle health and provide essential nutrients. Options like skinless chicken, fish, tofu, or well-cooked eggs are typically well-tolerated by individuals with gastroparesis.

e) Nut butters: Smooth and creamy nut butters, such as almond or peanut butter, can provide a good source of healthy fats and proteins. Spread them on toast or incorporate them into smoothies for added flavor and nutrition.

Remember, individual tolerance to foods can vary. It is essential to listen to your body and identify which specific foods work best for you. Keep a food diary and note how different foods make you feel to create a personalized list of safe and well-tolerated options.

4.2 High-Fiber Foods for Gastroparesis

While a gastroparesis diet typically limits high-fiber foods, it is still important to incorporate some fiber into your meals to support overall digestion and bowel regularity. However, the key is to choose soluble fibers, which are easier to digest compared to insoluble fibers.

Here are some high-fiber foods that are generally well-tolerated by individuals with gastroparesis:

a) Cooked and pureed vegetables: Vegetables that are cooked until soft and then pureed can provide a good source of soluble fiber. Options like pureed carrots, pumpkin, or spinach can be added to soups, sauces, or smoothies.

b) Oatmeal: Cooked oatmeal is a nutritious and high-fiber option that can be well-tolerated by individuals with gastroparesis. Opt for plain or flavored oatmeal without added fruits or nuts, as these can increase the fiber content and may be harder to digest.

c) Chia seeds: Chia seeds are a fantastic source of soluble fiber and can be added to yogurt, pudding, or smoothies. These tiny seeds absorb liquid and form a gel-like consistency, which can aid in digestion.

d) Applesauce: Unsweetened applesauce provides soluble fiber and is typically well-tolerated. Choose applesauce without added sugars or chunks of fruit for easier digestion.

Remember, individual tolerance to fiber can vary. It is crucial to introduce high-fiber foods slowly and monitor how they affect your symptoms. If you experience discomfort or increased symptoms, it may be necessary to reduce or avoid high-fiber foods.

4.3 Lean Proteins and Plant-Based Options

Protein is an essential macronutrient that plays a crucial role in supporting muscle health, promoting satiety, and providing essential amino acids for various bodily functions. Including lean proteins in your gastroparesis diet can help ensure you meet your nutritional needs.

Here are some lean protein options that are generally well-tolerated:

a) Skinless chicken or turkey: Chicken or turkey breast without the skin is a lean source of protein. Opt for baked, grilled, or poached preparations for easier digestion.

b) Fish: Fish, such as salmon, trout, or cod, provides lean protein and is rich in omega-3 fatty acids. Choose mild-tasting fish that is well-cooked and easily flaked.

c) Tofu: Tofu is a plant-based protein source that is often well-tolerated by individuals with gastroparesis. Opt for silken tofu or softer varieties and incorporate them into stir-fries, soups, or smoothies.

d) Eggs: Eggs are a versatile and easily digestible source of protein. Cook them in various ways, such as boiled, poached, or scrambled, to find the preparation that suits you best.

e) Yogurt: Plain, low-fat yogurt can be a good source of protein and probiotics. Choose yogurt without added fruits or granola, as these can increase the fiber content and may be harder to digest.

Incorporating lean proteins into your meals helps provide essential nutrients while minimizing symptoms associated with gastroparesis. Experiment with different protein sources and cooking methods to find options that work best for you.

4.4 Healthy Fats and Oils

Healthy fats play a crucial role in overall health and should be included in a gastroparesis diet in moderation. They provide essential fatty acids, support vitamin absorption, and help promote satiety.

Here are some healthy fats and oils to incorporate into your gastroparesis diet:

a) Olive oil: Extra virgin olive oil is a heart-healthy option that can be used for cooking, salad dressings, or drizzling over roasted vegetables. It is rich in monounsaturated fats and has anti-inflammatory properties.

b) Avocado: Avocado is a nutrient-dense fruit that provides healthy fats, fiber, and essential vitamins. Mash it up and spread it on toast, add it to smoothies, or incorporate it into salads for a creamy and nutritious boost.

c) Nuts and seeds: Small portions of nuts and seeds can provide healthy fats and additional nutrients. Opt for options like almonds, walnuts, or flaxseeds, and ensure they are well-chewed or blended for easier digestion.

d) Nut butters: Smooth and creamy nut butters, such as almond or peanut butter, are excellent sources of healthy fats. Spread them on toast, add them to smoothies, or use them as a dip for fruits or vegetables.

Remember, while healthy fats are beneficial, moderation is key. Fats are calorie-dense, so it is essential to consume them in appropriate portions to maintain a balanced diet and manage symptoms effectively.

4.5   Incorporating   Fruits   and Vegetables

Fruits and vegetables are vital components of a healthy diet, providing essential vitamins, minerals, and fiber. While some individuals with gastroparesis may have difficulty digesting raw or high-fiber varieties, there are ways to incorporate fruits and vegetables that are well-tolerated.

Here are some tips for incorporating fruits and vegetables into your gastroparesis

diet:

a) Cooked and pureed vegetables: Cooking vegetables until they are soft and then pureeing them can make them easier to digest. Consider pureed carrots, pumpkin, or spinach, which can be added to soups, sauces, or smoothies.

b) Soft fruits: Choose fruits that are gentle on the stomach, such as bananas, melons, and cooked apples. These fruits provide essential vitamins and minerals while being easier to digest compared to their raw counterparts.

c) Fruit and vegetable juices: Juicing fruits and vegetables can remove the fiber and make them easier to digest. However, it's important to note that juices may cause blood sugar spikes in individuals with diabetes, so moderation and monitoring are key.

d) Blended smoothies: Blending fruits and vegetables into smoothies can provide a nutrient-dense and easily digestible option. Opt for well-blended smoothies without added fibers or seeds, which can increase the fiber content and may be harder to digest.

e) Canned or cooked fruits: Canned fruits, particularly those packed in their own juices, can be well-tolerated. Additionally, lightly cooking fruits can make them softer and more easily digested.

Remember, individual tolerance to fruits and vegetables can vary. It is important to introduce them slowly, monitor your symptoms, and identify which specific options work best for you. Keep a food diary and note how different fruits and vegetables make you feel to create a personalized list of well-tolerated options.

Incorporating a variety of safe and well-tolerated foods into your gastroparesis diet can ensure that you receive the necessary nutrients while managing your symptoms effectively. Stay open-minded, experiment with different preparations and combinations, and consult with your healthcare team or registered dietitian for personalized guidance.

In the next chapter, we will delve into the foods that should be avoided or limited in a gastroparesis diet. Understanding these culprits and making informed choices will further empower you in managing your symptoms and optimizing your overall well-being.

Get ready to explore the flip side of the gastroparesis diet and learn how to navigate potential triggers effectively. Remember, with knowledge and dedication, you can create a diet that supports your health and allows you to enjoy delicious and nourishing meals.

Chapter 5: Foods to Avoid or Limit with Gastroparesis

Welcome to Chapter 5 of our comprehensive guide on managing gastroparesis with a healthy diet. In this chapter, we will explore the foods that should be avoided or limited in a gastroparesis diet. Understanding these culprits and making informed choices will empower you to manage your symptoms effectively and optimize your overall well-being.

5.1 Foods That May Worsen Gastroparesis Symptoms

Certain foods have the potential to exacerbate symptoms of gastroparesis by causing delayed gastric emptying, increasing bloating, or triggering discomfort. While individual tolerances can vary, it is generally recommended to avoid or limit the following foods:

a) High-fat foods: Foods that are high in fat, such as fried foods, fatty cuts of meat, and full-fat dairy products, can be challenging to digest and may delay gastric emptying. These foods can also contribute to feelings of fullness, bloating, and discomfort.

b) High-fiber foods: Fiber is an essential component of a healthy diet, but for individuals with gastroparesis, high-fiber foods can be difficult to digest and may worsen symptoms. Examples of high-fiber foods to limit or avoid include whole grains, raw vegetables, and legumes.

c) Tough or fibrous meats: Meats that are tough or have a high connective tissue content, such as beef or pork roasts, can be harder to break down and may cause discomfort. Opt for lean and tender meats, like skinless chicken or fish, which are generally better tolerated.

d) Raw fruits and vegetables: Raw fruits and vegetables can be challenging to digest for individuals with gastroparesis. The high fiber content and the tough texture can contribute to delayed gastric emptying and increased bloating.

Consider cooking or pureeing fruits and vegetables to make them easier to digest.

e) Carbonated beverages: Carbonated beverages, including soda and sparkling water, can contribute to feelings of bloating and discomfort. The bubbles in these drinks can increase gas production in the stomach, leading to distension and exacerbating symptoms.

5.2 Common Culprits for Delayed Gastric Emptying

Delayed gastric emptying is a hallmark of gastroparesis, and certain foods have been identified as common culprits that can further slow down the emptying process. It is important to be aware of these foods and consider limiting or avoiding them to help manage your symptoms effectively.

a) High-fat foods: As mentioned earlier, high-fat foods take longer to digest, which can lead to delayed gastric emptying. Fried foods, fatty cuts of meat, creamy sauces, and full-fat dairy products are examples of high-fat foods that may contribute to slower digestion.

b) High-fiber foods: While fiber is beneficial for overall health, excessive fiber intake can worsen symptoms of gastroparesis. Whole grains, raw vegetables, bran, and seeds are examples of high-fiber foods that can contribute to delayed gastric emptying.

c) Spicy foods: Spicy foods, such as chili peppers, hot sauces, and spicy seasonings, can irritate the stomach lining and potentially slow down digestion. For individuals with gastroparesis, it may be helpful to limit or avoid these foods to prevent discomfort and delayed gastric emptying.

d) Caffeine and alcohol: Both caffeine and alcohol can affect stomach motility and contribute to delayed gastric emptying. It is advisable to limit or avoid caffeinated beverages like coffee, tea, and energy drinks, as well as alcoholic beverages.

5.3 Managing Sugar and Sweeteners

For individuals with gastroparesis who also have diabetes or struggle with blood sugar control, managing sugar and sweeteners is crucial. It is important to be mindful of the impact of sugary foods on blood sugar levels and consider alternative sweeteners that are better tolerated.

a) Sugary foods and beverages: Foods and beverages high in added sugars can cause rapid spikes in blood sugar levels, which can be challenging to manage for individuals with diabetes and gastroparesis. Limit or avoid sugary snacks, candies, sodas, and desserts.

b) Artificial sweeteners: Some individuals with gastroparesis may find certain artificial sweeteners, such as sorbitol, mannitol, and xylitol, to exacerbate symptoms like bloating and diarrhea. It is advisable to monitor your tolerance to these sweeteners and consider alternatives like stevia or monk fruit extract.

c) Natural sweeteners: Natural sweeteners like honey, maple syrup, and agave nectar can be alternatives to refined sugars. However, it is important to use these sweeteners in moderation and monitor their impact on blood sugar levels.

5.4 Alcohol and Caffeine Considerations

Alcohol and caffeine are commonly consumed substances that can impact digestion and exacerbate symptoms of gastroparesis. While individual tolerances can vary, it is advisable to exercise caution and be mindful of their effects.

a) Alcohol: Alcohol can affect stomach motility and delay gastric emptying. It can also interact with medications commonly used to manage gastroparesis, leading to adverse effects. It is generally recommended to limit or avoid alcohol consumption.

b) Caffeine: Caffeine is a stimulant that can affect stomach contractions and potentially slow down gastric emptying. Limit or avoid caffeinated beverages like coffee, tea, energy drinks, and colas. Opt for caffeine-free alternatives or herbal teas instead.

Understanding the impact of certain foods, sugar and sweeteners, alcohol, and caffeine on gastroparesis symptoms empowers you to make informed choices and better manage your condition. It is important to listen to your body, monitor your individual tolerances, and work closely with your healthcare team or registered dietitian to develop a personalized plan that meets your specific needs.

In the next chapter, we will explore meal plans and recipes specifically designed for individuals with gastroparesis. These practical resources will provide inspiration and guidance on creating delicious and well-tolerated meals that support your journey towards managing gastroparesis effectively.

Stay motivated and continue to educate yourself on the best ways to nourish your body while managing your symptoms. You have the power to take control of your diet and live a fulfilling life despite the challenges of gastroparesis.

Chapter 6: Gastroparesis-Friendly Meal Plans and Recipes

Welcome to Chapter 6 of our comprehensive guide on managing gastroparesis with a healthy diet. In this chapter, we will explore meal plans and recipes specifically designed for individuals with gastroparesis. These practical resources will provide inspiration and guidance on creating delicious and well-tolerated meals that support your journey towards managing gastroparesis effectively.

6.1 The Importance of Meal Planning with Gastroparesis

Meal planning is a valuable tool for individuals with gastroparesis as it helps ensure that you have appropriate foods on hand and can make informed choices to manage your symptoms effectively. By planning your meals in advance, you can take control of your diet, optimize your nutrient intake, and reduce the stress of deciding what to eat each day.

Here are some key benefits of meal planning for gastroparesis:

a) Consistency and routine: Establishing a consistent eating schedule can help regulate stomach motility and improve digestion. Meal planning allows you to space out your meals and snacks evenly throughout the day, providing a sense of routine that can benefit your digestive system.

b) Portion control and balanced nutrition: By planning your meals in advance, you can ensure that you are consuming appropriate portion sizes and incorporating a variety of nutrients into your diet. This promotes optimal digestion and helps you meet your nutritional needs.

c) Grocery shopping efficiency: Meal planning enables you to create a well-thought-out shopping list, reducing the risk of impulse purchases and ensuring that you have the necessary ingredients for your gastroparesis-friendly meals.

d) Reduced food waste: Planning your meals allows you to use ingredients efficiently and minimize food waste. By purchasing only what you need and incorporating leftovers into future meals, you can make the most out of your ingredients and reduce unnecessary waste.

6.2 Building a Gastroparesis-Friendly Meal Plan

When creating a gastroparesis-friendly meal plan, it is important to consider your individual tolerances, preferences, and nutritional needs. Working closely with a registered dietitian or nutritionist can provide valuable guidance and ensure that your meal plan is tailored to your specific requirements.

Here are some key principles to keep in mind when building a gastroparesis-friendly meal plan:

a) Smaller, more frequent meals: Aim for 5-6 smaller meals spaced evenly throughout the day. This helps reduce the workload on your stomach and promotes better digestion.

b) Balanced meals: Include a variety of nutrients in each meal to ensure balanced nutrition. Incorporate lean proteins, cooked vegetables, low-fiber grains, and healthy fats into your meals.

c) Soft and well-cooked foods: Choose foods that are soft, tender, and well-cooked. These are generally easier to digest and less likely to cause discomfort. Consider pureed or mashed options to further aid digestion.

d) Mindful portion control: Pay attention to portion sizes and listen to your body's hunger and fullness cues. Eat until you feel comfortably satisfied, rather than overeating or forcing yourself to finish a large portion.

e) Fluid intake: Stay adequately hydrated by sipping water throughout the day. Consider incorporating hydrating foods like clear broths, herbal teas, and fruits with high water content.

Remember, individual tolerances and preferences can vary. Modify the meal plan according to your specific needs and work with your healthcare team or registered dietitian for personalized guidance.

6.3 Sample Gastroparesis-Friendly Meal Plan

To provide you with a starting point, here is a sample gastroparesis-friendly meal plan for a day:

Breakfast:

- Smoothie made with 1 cup of lactose-free yogurt, ½ cup of cooked and pureed fruit (such as applesauce or banana), 1 tablespoon of almond butter, and a handful of spinach.

- 2 slices of white toast with a thin spread of butter or a small amount of jam.

Snack:

- 1 small cup of low-fat cottage cheese.

Lunch:

- Grilled chicken breast (3-4 ounces) seasoned with herbs and served with a side of well-cooked mashed sweet potatoes.

- Cooked carrots or green beans.

Snack:

- 1 small ripe banana.

Dinner:

- Baked or broiled white fish (such as tilapia or cod) seasoned with lemon juice and herbs, served with a side of white rice.

- Steamed or lightly cooked zucchini or squash.

Snack:

- 1 small cup of lactose-free yogurt.

Before bed:

- 1 cup of chamomile tea.

Note: Remember to modify the portion sizes and food choices based on your specific needs and tolerances. Consult with your healthcare team or registered dietitian for personalized recommendations.

6.4 Gastroparesis-Friendly Recipe Ideas

Here are some gastroparesis-friendly recipe ideas to inspire you and add variety to your meal plan:

1. Creamy Butternut Squash Soup:

- Ingredients: Butternut squash, low-sodium chicken or vegetable broth, onion, garlic, nutmeg, salt, and pepper.

- Instructions: Roast the butternut squash, then blend it with the broth, onion, garlic, and seasonings until smooth. Heat the mixture on the stove until warmed through, adjusting the consistency with additional broth if desired.

2. Turkey and Vegetable Stir-Fry:

- Ingredients: Lean ground turkey, mixed vegetables (such as bell peppers, zucchini, and carrots), low-sodium soy sauce, garlic, ginger, and sesame oil.

- Instructions: Cook the ground turkey in a non-stick pan, then add the vegetables, soy sauce, garlic, ginger, and sesame oil. Stir-fry until the vegetables are tender and the flavors are well combined.

3. Baked Salmon with Lemon and Dill:

- Ingredients: Salmon fillet, lemon juice, fresh dill, salt, and pepper.

- Instructions: Place the salmon on a baking sheet, drizzle with lemon juice, and sprinkle with fresh dill, salt, and pepper. Bake in the oven until the salmon is cooked through and flakes easily with a fork.

4. Smoothie Bowl:

- Ingredients: Frozen berries, spinach, almond milk, chia seeds, and a topping of sliced bananas, shredded coconut, and a sprinkle of granola.

- Instructions: Blend the frozen berries, spinach, almond milk, and chia seeds until smooth. Pour the mixture into a bowl and top with sliced bananas, shredded coconut, and a sprinkle of granola for added texture.

Remember, these are just a few examples, and you can modify them based on your individual preferences and tolerances. Experiment with different ingredients, cooking methods, and seasonings to create meals that are both delicious and well-tolerated.

Incorporating a variety of gastroparesis-friendly meals and recipes into your diet ensures that you have an enjoyable culinary experience while managing your symptoms effectively.

In the final chapter, we will discuss the importance of emotional well-being and support in navigating life with gastroparesis. We will explore coping strategies, lifestyle modifications, and resources that can help you thrive despite the challenges. Prepare yourself for valuable insights and empowering guidance that will contribute to your overall well-being.

Gastroparesis is a condition that affects the normal spontaneous movement of the muscles (motility) in your stomach. Ordinarily, strong muscular contractions propel food through your digestive tract. But if you have gastroparesis, your stomach's motility is slowed down or doesn't work at all, preventing your stomach from emptying properly.

The cause of gastroparesis is usually unknown. Sometimes it's a complication of diabetes, and some people develop gastroparesis after surgery. Certain medications, such as opioid pain relievers, some antidepressants, and high blood pressure and allergy medications, can lead to slow gastric emptying and cause similar symptoms. For people who already have gastroparesis, these medications may make their condition worse.

Gastroparesis can interfere with normal digestion, cause nausea, vomiting and abdominal pain. It can also cause problems with blood sugar levels and nutrition. Although there's no cure for gastroparesis, changes to your diet, along with medication, can offer some relief.

Symptoms

Signs and symptoms of gastroparesis include:

• Vomiting

• Nausea

• Abdominal bloating

• Abdominal pain

• A feeling of fullness after eating just a few bites

• Vomiting undigested food eaten a few hours earlier

• Acid reflux

• Changes in blood sugar levels

• Lack of appetite

• Weight loss and malnutrition

Many people with gastroparesis don't have any noticeable signs and symptoms.

When to see a doctor

Make an appointment with your doctor if you have any signs or symptoms that worry you.

Causes

It's not always clear what leads to gastroparesis, but in some cases it can be caused by damage to a nerve that controls the stomach muscles (vagus nerve).

The vagus nerve helps manage the complex processes in your digestive tract, including signaling the muscles in your stomach to contract and push food into the small intestine. A damaged vagus nerve can't send signals normally to your stomach muscles. This may cause food to remain in your stomach longer, rather than move into your small intestine to be digested.

The vagus nerve and its branches can be damaged by diseases, such as diabetes, or by surgery to the stomach or small intestine.

Risk factors

Factors that can increase your risk of gastroparesis:

• Diabetes

• Abdominal or esophageal surgery

• Infection, usually from a virus

• Certain medications that slow the rate of stomach emptying, such as narcotic pain medications

• Scleroderma — a connective tissue disease

• Nervous system diseases, such as Parkinson's disease or multiple sclerosis

• Underactive thyroid (hypothyroidism)

Women are more likely to develop gastroparesis than are men.

Complications

Gastroparesis can cause several complications, such as:

• Severe dehydration. Ongoing vomiting can cause dehydration.

• Malnutrition. Poor appetite can mean you don't take in enough calories, or you may be unable to absorb enough nutrients due to vomiting.

• Undigested food that hardens and remains in your stomach. Undigested food in your stomach can harden into a solid mass called a bezoar. Bezoars can cause nausea and vomiting and may be life-threatening if they prevent food from passing into your small intestine.

• Unpredictable blood sugar changes. Although gastroparesis doesn't cause diabetes, frequent changes in the rate and amount of food passing into the small bowel can cause erratic changes in blood sugar levels. These variations in blood sugar make diabetes worse. In turn, poor control of blood sugar levels makes gastroparesis worse.

• Decreased quality of life. Symptoms can make it difficult to work and keep up with other responsibilities.

SHRIMP AND ARTICHOKE GREEN SALAD WITH LEMONY VINAIGRETTE

INGREDIENTS

GREEN SALAD INGREDIENTS:

- 1 batch Italian herb shrimp (see below)

- 1 batch Lemony Vinaigrette (see below)

- 5 ounces (about 5–6 cups) spring greens

- 2 cups diced tomatoes, cut into bite-sized pieces

- 1 (14 ounce) jar quartered artichoke hearts, drained and roughly chopped

- half of a small red onion, peeled and thinly-sliced

- 1/2 cup toasted pine nuts

- lots of freshly-grated Parmesan cheese

ITALIAN HERB SHRIMP INGREDIENTS:

- 8 ounces (1/2 pound) raw shrimp, peeled (or tail-on), deveined, and thawed

- 1 tablespoon Italian seasoning, store-bought or homemade

- salt and freshly-cracked black pepper

- 1 tablespoon extra-virgin olive oil

LEMONY VINAIGRETTE INGREDIENTS:

- 1/3 cup extra-virgin olive oil

- 3 tablespoons red wine vinegar

- 3 tablespoons freshly-squeezed lemon juice

- 1 teaspoon Italian seasoning, store-bought or homemade

- 1/2 teaspoon Kosher salt

- 1/2 teaspoon freshly-cracked black pepper

- 1 garlic clove, pressed or minced

- (optional: 1 teaspoon honey, if you'd like a sweeter dressing)

INSTRUCTIONS

TO MAKE THE GREEN SALAD:

1. Add all ingredients together in a large bowl, and toss until evenly combined. Serve immediately, garnished with extra Parmesan cheese and freshly-cracked black pepper if desired.

TO MAKE THE ITALIAN HERB SHRIMP:

1. Sprinkle shrimp evenly on both sides with the Italian seasoning, and a few generous pinches of salt and pepper.

2. Heat oil in a large saute pan over medium-high heat. Add shrimp and cook for 4-5 minutes, stirring and flipping occasionally, until the shrimp are pink and cooked through and no longer opaque. Remove from heat and serve immediately.

TO MAKE THE LEMONY VINAIGRETTE:

1. Whisk all ingredients together until combined.

KALE SALAD WITH BACON AND BLUE CHEESE

INGREDIENTS

KALE SALAD INGREDIENTS:

- 6–7 cups chopped fresh kale leaves

- 1 tablespoon Bertolli Extra Virgin Olive Oil

- 6–8 slices cooked bacon, chopped

- 1/2 cup crumbled blue cheese

- 1/2 cup dried cranberries

- 1/2 cup toasted chopped pecans

- 1 batch Red Wine Shallot Vinaigrette (below)

RED WINE SHALLOT VINAIGRETTE INGREDIENTS:

- 1/4 cup Bertolli Extra Virgin Olive Oil

- 2 tablespoons red wine vinegar

- 1–2 teaspoons honey, to taste

- 1 teaspoon Dijon mustard

- pinch of salt and freshly-cracked black pepper

- 1 small shallot, peeled and finely-chopped

INSTRUCTIONS

TO MAKE THE KALE SALAD:

1. Toss all ingredients together until combined.

2. Serve immediately, or cover and refrigerate for up to 8 hours before serving.

TO MAKE THE RED WINE SHALLOT VINAIGRETTE:

1. Whisk the olive oil, red wine vinegar, honey, mustard, salt and pepper together in a mixing bowl until completely combined. (Or you can toss everything in a mason jar and give it a good shake.) Stir in the shallot until combined. Taste, and season with extra salt and/or pepper and/or honey, if needed.

CUCUMBER QUINOA SALAD

INGREDIENTS

CUCUMBER QUINOA SALAD INGREDIENTS:

- 1 English cucumber, diced

- 2 cups chilled* cooked quinoa

- 1/2 cup diced red onion

- 1/2 cup crumbled feta cheese

- 1/3 cup julienned or roughly-chopped fresh basil leaves

- 1 batch Lemony Italian vinaigrette (see below)

LEMONY ITALIAN VINAIGRETTE INGREDIENTS:

- 1/4 cup olive oil

- 2 tablespoons apple cider vinegar or red wine vinegar

- 1 tablespoon fresh lemon juice

- 1/2 teaspoon Italian seasoning, homemade or store-bought

- pinch of salt and black pepper

INSTRUCTIONS

TO MAKE THE CUCUMBER QUINOA SALAD:

1. Toss all ingredients together until combined. Serve immediately.

TO MAKE THE LEMONY ITALIAN VINAIGRETTE:

1. Whisk all ingredients together in a small bowl until combined.

NOTES

*If you add hot quinoa fresh out of the pan, it will melt the cheese and wilt the basil a bit in this recipe. So I recommend cooking it beforehand and letting it chill in the refrigerator before making the salad. Or, if you need to cook it immediately beforehand, just spread the cooked quinoa out in a thin layer on a baking sheet and pop it in the freezer for 15-20 minutes. That will help it cool down nice and quickly!

TABBOULEH

INGREDIENTS

- 1/2 cup uncooked bulgur

- 2 cups of chicken or vegetable stock

- 2–3 cups of chopped Italian flat-leaf parsley, loosely packed

- 1/2 cup of chopped mint

- 1/4 cup of chopped scallions

- 2–3 roma tomatoes, cored and chopped

- 2 tablespoons olive oil

- 2 tablespoons lemon juice

- 1/2 tsp salt

INSTRUCTIONS

1. In a large bowl, pour 2 cups of boiling water (or chicken stock) over the bulgur. Let it sit for 30-60 minutes until softened, and then strain the bulgur through a fine-mesh strainer.

2. Then combine the prepared bulgur, parsley, mint, scallions, and tomatoes in a large bowl. Add oil and lemon juice, and stir until well mixed. Add salt to taste.

3. Serve immediately or refrigerate for up to one day.

ARUGULA SALAD WITH PARMESAN, LEMON AND OLIVE OIL

INGREDIENTS

• 2 handfuls fresh baby arugula

• 2 Tablespoons freshly-grated Parmesan, plus extra shavings as garnish

• 2 teaspoons good-quality olive oil

• 2 teaspoons freshly-squeezed lemon juice

• 1 teaspoon freshly-cracked black pepper

INSTRUCTIONS

1. Add arugula and Parmesan to a large mixing bowl. Drizzle evenly with olive oil and lemon juice, and sprinkle with black pepper. Toss until combined.

2. Serve immediately, garnished with extra Parmesan if desired.

AVOCADO POTATO SALAD

INGREDIENTS

- 3 pounds Yukon Gold or red potatoes, quartered

- Kosher salt

- 2 Tablespoons ALDI SimplyNature apple cider vinegar

- 1 1/4 cups ALDI FriendlyFarms plain Greek yogurt or mayonnaise

- 1 tablespoon Dijon mustard

- 1/4 teaspoon freshly-cracked black pepper

- 4 hard-boiled eggs, peeled and diced

- 2 medium organic avocados, peeled, pitted and diced

- half of a small red onion, peeled and thinly-sliced (or diced)

- 1/2 cup chopped celery (about 2–3 celery ribs)

- 1/4 cup chopped fresh cilantro

• optional toppings: pinch of chili powder, extra chopped fresh cilantro, extra black pepper

INSTRUCTIONS

1. Place the potatoes in the bottom of a large stockpot. Fill the pot with cold water until it reaches an inch above the potatoes, then add a tablespoon of salt to the water.

2. Heat the potatoes over high heat until the water reaches a rolling boil. Then reduce heat to medium, and simmer for 15-20 minutes, or until the potatoes are fork-tender and cooked through.

3. Remove from heat and strain out the water. Then once the potatoes have cooled for a few minutes, remove and discard the potato skins. Then dice the potatoes into small bite-sized pieces, and sprinkle with the vinegar. Set aside.

4. In a large mixing bowl, whisk together the Greek yogurt (or mayo), Dijon mustard and black pepper until combined.

5. Add the diced potatoes, hard-boiled eggs, avocado, red onion, celery and cilantro to the mixing bowl. Then very gently toss the potato salad until all of the ingredients are combined and evenly coated with the Greek yogurt sauce.

6. Garnish with optional toppings if desired.

7. Serve immediately. Or cover the salad with plastic wrap so that the plastic is completely touching the top of the salad with no air bubbles, and refrigerate for up to 2 days. (The avocados may brown slightly after a few hours, but they will still be safe and delicious to eat.)

GREEN SALAD WITH BEETS, ORANGES & AVOCADO

INGREDIENTS

- 4 cups leafy greens (I used a chard/kale/arugula/spinach mix)

- 3 small oranges, peeled and sliced into rounds

- 1 avocado, peeled, pitted and diced

- 1 large carrot, peeled and julienned

- 1 small beet, peeled and julienned

- 1/2 cup crumbled feta or goat cheese

- 1/4 cup toasted pepitas

- 1/3 cup white balsamic vinaigrette (or any vinaigrette)

INSTRUCTIONS

1. Add greens, oranges, avocado, carrot, beets, pepitas, and cheese together in a large bowl. Drizzle evenly with the vinaigrette, and toss until the salad is combined and evenly coated.

2. Serve immediately, topped with some freshly-cracked black pepper if desired.

GREEK YOGURT COLESLAW

INGREDIENTS

- 1 (10-ounce) bag shredded cabbage (about 4 cups)*

- 1 cup shredded carrots

- 1/2 cup thinly-sliced green onions

- 2/3 cups non-fat plain Greek yogurt

- 1 tablespoon lemon juice

- 2 Tablespoons apple cider vinegar

- 2 Tablespoons honey, warmed

- 1 teaspoon Dijon mustard (optional)

- 1/4 tsp celery salt

- pinch of salt and freshly-cracked black pepper

INSTRUCTIONS

1. Combine the cabbage, carrot and green onions in a large bow, and toss to combine.

2. In a separate bowl, whisk together Greek yogurt, lemon juice, vinegar, honey, mustard celery salt, and a pinch of salt and pepper until combine. Taste, and season with extra salt and pepper if needed.

3. Pour the Greek yogurt mixture into the cabbage mixture, and toss until evenly combined.

4. Serve immediately, or cover and refrigerate for up to 4 hours.

ROASTED BUTTERNUT SQUASH, KALE AND CRANBERRY COUSCOUS

INGREDIENTS

COUSCOUS SALAD INGREDIENTS:

• 1 small butternut squash, peeled, seeded, and diced into 1/2-inch cubes

• 2 tablespoons olive oil

• salt and freshly-cracked black pepper

• 1 cup dry Israeli (pearl) couscous*, cooked in water according to package instructions

• 2 cups chopped kale leaves

• 1/3 cup dried cranberries

• 1/3 cup chopped walnuts

• 2 ounces goat cheese, crumbled

• easy orange vinaigrette (recipe below)

VINAIGRETTE INGREDIENTS:

• 2 tablespoons apple cider vinegar

• 2 tablespoons DeLallo extra virgin olive oil

• 2 tablespoons freshly-squeezed orange juice

• pinch of salt and black pepper, to taste

INSTRUCTIONS

TO MAKE THE COUSCOUS SALAD:

1. Heat oven to 425°F.

2. In a large mixing bowl, toss cubed butternut squash with olive oil. Sprinkle with a few generous pinches of salt and pepper, and toss until combined.

3. Spread the butternut squash out in an even layer on a parchment-covered baking sheet. Bake for 15 minutes, then remove from the oven and flip the squash for even cooking. Bake for an additional 10-15 minutes, or until the squash is tender and slightly browned around the edges.

Remove from oven and transfer back to the large mixing bowl.

4. Add couscous, kale, cranberries, walnuts, goat cheese, and vinaigrette, and toss to combine.

5. Serve warm, or refrigerate in a sealed container for up to 3 days.

TO MAKE THE VINAGIRETTE:

1. Whisk all ingredients together until combined. Taste, and season with additional salt and pepper if needed.

KALE CAESAR SALAD

INGREDIENTS

KALE CAESAR SALAD INGREDIENTS:

• 4 cups chopped fresh kale

• 4 cups chopped Romaine lettuce

• 2 cups croutons (*I just toasted some French bread and crumbled it afterwards, see instructions below)

- 3/4 cup grated Parmesan cheese

- 1 batch Lime Caesar Dressing, below

- optional: 1 cup halved cherry or grape tomatoes

LIME CAESAR DRESSING INGREDIENTS:

- 1/2 cup plain Greek yogurt (I used non-fat)

- 1/2 cup freshly-grated Parmesan cheese

- 3–4 tablespoons fresh lime juice

- 1 tablespoon extra-virgin olive oil

- 1–2 teaspoons anchovy paste, to taste

- 2 teaspoons worcestershire sauce

- 1 clove garlic, pressed or finely minced

- 1 teaspoon Dijon mustard

- 1/4 teaspoon sea salt

- pinch of black pepper

- 3–4 tablespoons milk

INSTRUCTIONS

TO MAKE THE KALE CAESAR SALAD:

1. Add the kale, Romaine, croutons, Parmesan, dressing, and tomatoes (if using) to a large bowl. Toss until combined.

2. Serve immediately.

TO MAKE THE LIME CAESAR DRESSING:

1. Add all ingredients except milk to a small mixing bowl, and whisk together until combined and smooth. Whisk in a tablespoon of milk at a time until the dressing reaches your desired consistency.

2. Use immediately, or refrigerate in a sealed container for up to 3 days.

NOTES

*To make easy croutons, just drizzle a few slices of old bread with olive oil (or brush with melted butter), and sprinkle with salt and Italian seasoning. Toast them up until crispy. Then either crumble them up with your hands, or use a knife to chop them into small pieces.

MEDITERRANEAN FARRO SALAD

INGREDIENTS

SALAD INGREDIENTS:

- 3 cups chicken or vegetable stock

- 1 cup uncooked farro, rinsed and drained

- 1 large cucumber, seeded and finely-diced

- 2/3 cup finely-diced roasted red peppers

- 1/2 cup finely-diced sun-dried tomatoes

- 1/2 cup crumbled feta cheese

- half of a small red onion, finely diced (about 2/3 cup)

- 1/4 cup finely-chopped fresh parsley

- Greek vinaigrette (see ingredients below)

Greek Vinaigrette Ingredients:

- 3 Tablespoons olive oil

- 1 Tablespoon freshly-squeezed lemon juice

- 1 Tablespoon red wine vinegar

- 1/4 teaspoon dried oregano

- pinch of garlic powder

- pinch of salt

- pinch of black pepper

INSTRUCTIONS

TO MAKE THE SALAD:

1. Stir together stock and farro in a medium saucepan, and cook according to package instructions until al dente. Remove from heat, and drain off any extra stock once the farro is cooked. Let farro cool for at least 10 minutes.

2. Transfer farro to a large mixing bowl, and add in remaining ingredients, including the vinaigrette. Toss until combined.

3. Serve immediately, or cover and refrigerate for up to 2 days.

TO MAKE THE GREEK VINAIGRETTE:

1. Whisk all ingredients together until combined. Use immediately.

SESAME QUINOA SALAD

INGREDIENTS

SLAW INGREDIENTS:

- 1 (16-ounce) bag shredded red cabbage (or about 4 cups shredded cabbage)

- 2 cups cooked quinoa (I used red quinoa)

- 2 cups shredded carrots

- 2/3 cup thinly-sliced green onions

- 1/2 cup slivered or sliced almonds, toasted

- 2 tablespoons sesame seeds

SESAME HONEY VINAIGRETTE INGREDIENTS:

- 1/3 cup vegetable oil (or any cooking oil)

- 3 Tablespoons rice wine vinegar

- 1 tablespoon honey (or agave, to make this vegan)

- 1 teaspoon soy sauce

- 1/8 teaspoon sesame oil

- pinch of salt and black pepper

INSTRUCTIONS

TO MAKE THE SLAW:

1. Toss all ingredients together until combined. Serve immediately, or refrigerate in a sealed container for up to 1 day.

TO MAKE THE ASIAN HONEY VINAIGRETTE:

1. Whisk all ingredients together until combined.

CAESAR SALAD RECIPE

INGREDIENTS

- 1 head of Romaine lettuce

- 2 cups croutons, homemade or store-bought

- 1 batch Greek yogurt Caesar dressing

- 1/4 cup freshly-grated Parmesan cheese*, plus more for topping

INSTRUCTIONS

1. Toss the Romaine, croutons, Greek yogurt Caesar dressing and 1/4 cup Parmesan cheese together until combined. Serve immediately, topped with extra Parmesan cheese.

WHITE BALSAMIC VINAIGRETTE

INGREDIENTS

• 1/2 cup DeLallo extra virgin olive oil

• 1/4 cup DeLallo Golden Balsamic Vinegar (a.k.a. "white" balsamic vinegar)

• 2–3 tablespoons honey or agave or desired sweetener

• 1/2 teaspoon sea salt

• 1/4 teaspoon freshly-cracked black pepper

• 1/4 teaspoon Italian seasoning (store-bought or homemade)

INSTRUCTIONS

1. Whisk all ingredients together for 30 seconds or until blended.

POMEGRANATE, PEAR AND AVOCADO SALAD

INGREDIENTS

SALAD INGREDIENTS:

• 1 head Romaine lettuce, washed and roughly-chopped into bite-sized pieces

• 1 ripe pear, cored and diced

• 1 avocado, peeled, pitted and diced

• 2/3 cup shelled pistachios

• 2/3 cup crumbled goat cheese (or blue cheese, or feta cheese)

• 1/2 cup diced red onion (about half of a small red onion)

• seeds from 1 pomegranate (here is a tutorial for how to open and de-seed a pomegranate)

• citrus vinaigrette (see below)

CITRUS VINAIGRETTE INGREDIENTS:

* 1/3 cup orange juice (freshly-squeezed, if possible)

* 1/4 cup white balsamic vinegar (or white wine vinegar)

* 1 tablespoon honey, if needed to sweeten

* 1/2 teaspoon kosher salt

* 1/4 teaspoon freshly-ground black pepper

* 1/3 cup olive oil

INSTRUCTIONS

TO MAKE THE SALAD:

1. Add all ingredients together in a large bowl and drizzle on the dressing. Toss until combined. Serve immediately.

2. (*Tip: To prevent the diced avocado from browning while sitting out, toss it beforehand in a few tablespoons of lime or lemon juice.)

TO MAKE THE VINAIGRETTE:

1. Whisk all ingredients together for 30 seconds until combined.

FUJI APPLE CHICKEN SALAD

INGREDIENTS

SALAD INGREDIENTS:

- 1 Tbsp. extra virgin olive oil

- 2 boneless, skinless chicken breasts

- 1 (10 oz.) bag mixed greens

- quarter of a red onion, thinly sliced

- 2 cups apple chips

- 1 cup glazed pecans

- 1/2 cup gorgonzola cheese, crumbled

- 1 cup freshly-diced tomatoes (optional)

WHITE BALSAMIC VINAIGRETTE INGREDIENTS:

- 1/2 cup extra virgin olive oil

- 1/4 cup white balsamic vinegar

- 2–3 tablespoons honey

- 1/2 teaspoon sea salt

- 1/4 teaspoon freshly-cracked black pepper

- 1/8 teaspoon garlic powder

INSTRUCTIONS

TO MAKE THE SALAD:

1. Preheat oven to 350 degrees F. Prepare a baking sheet with aluminum foil, then mist it with cooking spray or oil.

2. Brush chicken breasts with olive oil, then season with a pinch of salt and freshly ground black pepper. (Or you can add your favorite seasonings.) Place on prepared baking sheet, and cook for 20-30 minutes, or until internal temperature is 160 degrees and the juices run clear. Remove and let chicken cool for at least 10 minutes, then thinly slice or shred.

3. Toss the remaining salad ingredients together in a large bowl, and drizzle on your desired

amount of vinaigrette. Toss and serve immediately.

TO MAKE THE VINAIGRETTE:

1. Whisk all ingredients together until blended.

CHOPPED KALE GREEK SALAD

INGREDIENTS

GREEK SALAD INGREDIENTS:

- 1 large bunch (about 10 ounces) kale leaves, finely chopped

- 1 pint cherry or grape tomatoes, halved

- 1 cucumber, seeded and diced

- 1 (15-ounce) can garbanzo beans (chickpeas), rinsed and drained

- 1/2 red onion, thinly sliced

- 2/3 cup Kalamata olives, pitted

- 2/3 cup crumbled feta cheese

- garlic parsley vinaigrette (see below)

GARLIC PARSLEY VINAIGRETTE INGREDIENTS:

- 1/2 cup olive oil

- 1/4 cup fresh parsley leaves, finely chopped

- 3 Tbsp. freshly-squeezed lemon juice

- 3 Tbsp. red wine vinegar

- 2 garlic cloves, pressed (or finely chopped)

- 1 tsp. dried oregano

- 1/2 tsp. sugar

- 1/4 tsp. salt

- 1/4 tsp. black pepper

INSTRUCTIONS

TO MAKE THE GREEK SALAD:

1. Toss all ingredients together with desired amount of dressing until evenly mixed.

TO MAKE THE GARLIC LEMON VINAIGRETTE:

1. Whisk all ingredients together until blended. Season with additional salt and pepper if needed.

GERMAN POTATO SALAD

INGREDIENTS

- 2 pounds Yukon gold potatoes

- 8 thick slices bacon

- half a large yellow onion, peeled and thinly sliced

- 1/3 cup apple cider vinegar

- 1 teaspoon salt (plus extra for salting the potato water)

- 1/2 teaspoon coarsely-ground black pepper (or more, to taste)

- ¼ cup chopped fresh parsley leaves

INSTRUCTIONS

1. Add potatoes into a large stockpot and cover with cold water that extends at least 2 inches above the potatoes. Stir in a generous pinch of salt. Bring to a boil over medium-high heat. Reduce heat to medium, and continue cooking

until potatoes are tender when pierced with a fork, about 15–20 minutes.

2. Meanwhile, cook bacon in a large saute pan over medium heat until crisp, stirring occasionally, about 10-12 minutes. Transfer bacon with a slotted spoon to a plate that has been covered with paper towels, and later break it into small pieces. Reserve 1 tablespoon of bacon grease in the pan, and discard the rest. Add onions to the saute pan and cook in the reserved bacon grease for 5 minutes, stirring occasionally, until cooked and translucent. Remove from heat and transfer onions to the plate with the bacon.

3. When the potatoes are cooked, drain them and cut into 1-inch cubes. Add potatoes to your serving bowl, and top with the cooked bacon, onions, vinegar, salt, and pepper. Toss to combine. Serve topped with fresh parsley.

RAINBOW ANTIPASTO PASTA SALAD

INGREDIENTS

RAINBOW ANTIPASTO SALAD INGREDIENTS:

- 1 pound dry pasta (I used tri-color rotini)

- 4–6 cups chopped antipasto ingredients (I used diced salami, mozzarella, cherry tomatoes, olives, artichoke hearts, pepperoncini, roasted red peppers. See below for more ideas.*)

- 1 cup chopped fresh kale, massaged**

- quarter of a small red onion, peeled and thinly-sliced

- 1 batch Italian Herb Vinaigrette (see below)

ITALIAN HERB VINAIGRETTE INGREDIENTS:

- 1/3 cup extra-virgin olive oil

- 1/4 cup red-wine vinegar

- 2 teaspoons McCormick Italian Blend Herb Grinder Italian seasoning, or homemade

- 1/2 teaspoon Kosher salt

- 1/2 teaspoon freshly-cracked black pepper

- 1/4 teaspoon garlic powder

INSTRUCTIONS

TO MAKE THE ANTIPASTO PASTA SALAD:

1. Cook the pasta in a large stockpot of generously-salted water al dente according to package directions. Drain pasta and rinse under cold water for about 20-30 seconds until no longer hot.

2. In a large bowl, combine the cooked pasta, antipasto ingredients, kale, and onion. Drizzle the Italian Herb Vinaigrette on top, then toss to combine. Serve immediately, or cover and refrigerate for up to 3 days.

TO MAKE THE ITALIAN HERB VINAIGRETTE:

1. Whisk all ingredients together until combined.

LIGHTENED-UP CHICKEN SALAD

INGREDIENTS

- 4 cups diced cooked chicken

- 1 cup chopped celery

- 1 cup plain low-fat Greek yogurt

- 1 cup seedless grapes, halved

- 1 small shallot, peeled and finely-diced

- 1/2 cup toasted walnuts

- 1/3 cup dried cranberries or cherries

- 1 teaspoon worchestershire sauce

- 1/2 teaspoon freshly-cracked black pepper

- 1/4 teaspoon Kosher salt

INSTRUCTIONS

1. Add all ingredients to a large bowl, and toss until combined and evenly-coated.

2. Serve immediately, or refrigerate in a sealed container for up to 3 days.

LEMONY ARTICHOKE PASTA SALAD

INGREDIENTS

PASTA SALAD INGREDIENTS:

- 1 pound (16 ounces) uncooked pasta (I used gemelli)

- 1 tablespoon olive oil

- 1 bunch (about 1 pound) asparagus, chopped into bite-sized pieces

- 4 cloves garlic, peeled and thinly-sliced

- Kosher salt and freshly-cracked black pepper

- 1 (14 ounce) jar artichoke hearts, drained and roughly-chopped

- 2/3 cup freshly-crated Parmesan cheese, plus extra for serving

- 1/2 cup toasted pine nuts

- 1 batch Lemon Basil Vinaigrette (see below)

LEMON BASIL VINAIGRETTE INGREDIENTS:

- 1/4 cup olive oil

- 3 tablespoons freshly-squeezed lemon juice

- 3 tablespoons finely-chopped fresh basil leaves

- 2 tablespoons red wine vinegar

- 1/2 teaspoon Kosher salt

- 1/4 teaspoon freshly-cracked black pepper

INSTRUCTIONS

TO MAKE THE PASTA SALAD:

1. Cook the pasta in a large stockpot of generously-salted water until it is al dente, according to package directions. Drain pasta and rinse under cold water for about 20-30 seconds until no longer hot. Set aside.

2. Meanwhile, as the pasta water is heating and the pasta is cooking, heat oil in a large saute pan over medium-high heat. Add chopped asparagus, season with a generous pinch of salt and pepper, and stir to combine. Sauté for 3 minutes, stirring occasionally. Stir in sliced garlic, and continue sautéing the mixture for 1-2 minutes more, stirring occasionally, until the garlic is fragrant and the asparagus is tender but still slightly crisp on the inside. Remove from heat and set aside.

3. In a large bowl, combine the cooked pasta, asparagus mixture, artichoke hearts, Parmesan and toasted pine nuts. Drizzle evenly with the lemon basil vinaigrette, then toss to combine.

4. Serve immediately, garnished with extra Parmesan if desired. Or cover and refrigerate in a sealed container for up to 3 days.

TO MAKE THE LEMON BASIL VINAIGRETTE:

1. Whisk all ingredients together in a small bowl or measuring cup until combined.

CUCUMBER QUINOA SALAD

INGREDIENTS

CUCUMBER QUINOA SALAD INGREDIENTS:

- 1 English cucumber, diced

- 2 cups chilled* cooked quinoa (see this tutorial for how to cook quinoa)

- 1/2 cup diced red onion

- 1/2 cup crumbled feta cheese

- 1/3 cup julienned or roughly-chopped fresh basil leaves

- 1 batch Lemony Italian vinaigrette (see below)

LEMONY ITALIAN VINAIGRETTE INGREDIENTS:

- 1/4 cup olive oil

- 2 tablespoons apple cider vinegar or red wine vinegar

- 1 tablespoon fresh lemon juice

- 1/2 teaspoon Italian seasoning, homemade or store-bought

- pinch of salt and black pepper

INSTRUCTIONS

TO MAKE THE CUCUMBER QUINOA SALAD:

1. Toss all ingredients together until combined. Serve immediately.

TO MAKE THE LEMONY ITALIAN VINAIGRETTE:

1. Whisk all ingredients together in a small bowl until combined.

PIZZA PASTA SALAD

INGREDIENTS

PIZZA PASTA SALAD INGREDIENTS:

- 1 pound uncooked pasta (I used farfalle)

- 8 ounces mozzarella, diced

- 1 cup diced roma tomatoes

- 4–6 cups chopped pizza toppings (I used pepperoni, black olives, and sliced red onions)

- 1 batch Garlic-Oregano Vinaigrette (see below)

- optional toppings: freshly-grated Parmesan cheese, crushed red pepper flakes

GARLIC-OREGANO VINAIGRETTE:

- 1/3 cup extra-virgin olive oil

- 1/4 cup white wine vinegar (or red wine vinegar)

- 3 garlic cloves, peeled and pressed (or minced)

- 1/2 teaspoon dried oregano

- 1/2 teaspoon Kosher salt

- 1/2 teaspoon freshly-cracked black pepper

INSTRUCTIONS

TO MAKE THE PIZZA PASTA SALAD:

1. Cook the pasta in a large stockpot of generously-salted water al dente according to package directions. Drain pasta and rinse under cold water for about 20-30 seconds until no longer hot. Drain completely.

2. In a large bowl, combine the cooled pasta, mozzarella, tomatoes, and pizza toppings. Drizzle the vinaigrette on top, then toss to combine. Garnish with your desired toppings.

3. Serve immediately, or cover and refrigerate for up to 3 days.

TO MAKE THE GARLIC-OREGANO VINAIGRETTE:

1. Whisk all ingredients together until combined

BERRY FRUIT SALAD

INGREDIENTS

- 1 pound fresh strawberries, hulled and halved

- 8 ounces fresh bing cherries, pitted

- 8 ounces fresh blackberries

- 8 ounces fresh blueberries

- 8 ounces fresh raspberries

- 1/4 cup chopped fresh mint leaves

- 2 tablespoons fresh lemon juice

- 1 tablespoon honey

INSTRUCTIONS

1. Add the strawberries, cherries, blackberries, blueberries, raspberries, and chopped mint together in a large bowl. Set aside.

2. In a separate bowl, whisk together the lemon juice and honey until combined.

3. Pour it on top of the berries. Then gently toss the fruit salad until everything is evenly coated with the lemon mixture.

4. Serve immediately, or refrigerate in a sealed container for up to 3 days.

MEDITERRANEAN PASTA SALAD

INGREDIENTS

MEDITERRANEAN PASTA SALAD INGREDIENTS:

- 12 ounces dry pasta (I used farfalle)

- 1 English cucumber, diced

- 1 pint cherry or grape tomatoes, halved

- 2/3 cup sliced kalamata olives

- 4 ounces crumbled feta cheese

- half of a medium red onion, peeled and thinly sliced

LEMON-HERB VINAIGRETTE INGREDIENTS:

- 1/4 cup extra virgin olive oil

- 3 tablespoons red wine vinegar

- 1 tablespoon freshly-squeezed lemon juice

- 2 teaspoons dried oregano, minced

- 1 teaspoon honey (or your desired sweetener)

- 2 small garlic cloves, minced

- 1/4 teaspoon freshly-cracked black pepper

- 1/4 teaspoon salt

• pinch of crushed red pepper flakes

INSTRUCTIONS

TO MAKE THE MEDITERRANEAN PASTA SALAD:

1. Cook the pasta al dente in a large stockpot of generously-salted water according to package instructions. Drain pasta, then rinse under cold water for about 20-30 seconds until no longer hot. Transfer the pasta to a large mixing bowl.

2. Add cucumber, tomatoes, kalamata olives, feta cheese, and red onion to the mixing bowl, then drizzle all of the vinaigrette evenly on top. Toss until all of the ingredients are evenly coated with the dressing.

3. Serve immediately, garnished with extra feta and black pepper if desired.

TO MAKE THE LEMON-HERB VINAIGRETTE:

1. Whisk all ingredients together until combined.

CAPRESE PASTA SALAD

INGREDIENTS

CAPRESE PASTA SALAD INGREDIENTS:

- 1 pound dry pasta (any shape will do)

- 1 pint cherry or grape tomatoes (I used a combination of red/yellow cherry tomatoes)

- 1 (8 oz) ball of fresh mozzarella, diced (or you can use the brick of cheese)

- 1/3 cup julienned or shredded fresh basil leaves

- 1 batch balsamic vinaigrette (see below)

BALSAMIC VINAIGRETTE INGREDIENTS:

- 1/3 cup extra virgin olive oil

- 3 tablespoons balsamic vinegar

- 1 tablespoon honey

- 1/4 teaspoon sea salt

- 1/4 teaspoon freshly-cracked black pepper

- pinch of Italian seasonings (store-bought or homemade)

INSTRUCTIONS

TO MAKE THE CAPRESE PASTA SALAD:

1. Cook the pasta in a large stockpot of generously-salted water al dente according to package directions. Drain pasta and rinse under cold water for about 20-30 seconds until no longer hot.

2. In a large serving bowl, toss pasta with the remaining ingredients until combined.

3. Serve immediately, or refrigerate in a sealed container for up to 3 days.

TO MAKE THE BALSAMIC VINAIGRETTE:

1. Whisk all ingredients together until combined.

CRUNCHY RAMEN NOODLE SALAD

INGREDIENTS

SALAD INGREDIENTS:

• 1 (16-ounce) bag coleslaw mix

• 2 (3-ounce) packages of ramen noodles*, crumbled (you will not use the seasoning packet)

- 1 cup shelled and cooked edamame

- 1 avocado, peeled, pitted and diced

- 1 mango, peeled, pitted, and julienned (or diced)

- 1/2 cup thinly-sliced almonds

- 1/2 cup thinly-sliced green onions (scallions)

- Sesame honey vinaigrette (see ingredients below)

SESAME HONEY VINAIGRETTE

- 1/2 cup avocado oil (or vegetable oil, or any cooking oil)

- 1/4 cup honey (or your desired sweetener)

- 1/4 cup rice vinegar

- 2 teaspoons soy sauce

- 1/4 teaspoon toasted sesame oil

- pinch of salt and black pepper

INSTRUCTIONS

TO MAKE THE SALAD:

1. Heat oven to 425°F. Spread the crumbled ramen noodles and sliced almonds out on a baking sheet, and stir a bit to combine. Bake for about 5 minutes, or until the almonds and noodles are slightly toasted and golden. Remove baking sheet, and give the mixture a good stir to toss. Then return it to the oven and toast for an additional 3 minutes. Keep a very close eye on the mixture so that it does not burn. Remove and set aside.

2. Add ingredients (including the vinaigrette) together in a large bowl, and toss until combined.

3. Serve immediately, or cover and refrigerate for up to 3 days. (This salad is much better eaten the first day, as the noodles lose their "crunch" the longer it sits, and the avocado may brown a bit. Still, it's perfectly edible and enjoyable even after a few days!)

TO MAKE THE VINAIGRETTE:

1. Whisk all ingredients together until combined.

ASIAN CHICKEN CHOPPED SALAD

INGREDIENTS

SALAD INGREDIENTS:

• 2 boneless skinless chicken breasts, grilled and sliced (see below for optional marinade)

• 1 head Napa or green cabbage, thinly sliced

• 1 large avocado, peeled, pitted and thinly sliced

• 1 cup shredded carrots

• 2/3 cup roughly-chopped fresh cilantro leaves

• 1/3 cup toasted sliced or slivered almonds

• 1/3 cup thinly-sliced green onions

• 1 tablespoon toasted sesame seeds

• 1 batch creamy sesame-almond dressing (see below)

CREAMY SESAME-ALMOND DRESSING INGREDIENTS:

- 1/3 cup Blue Diamond Almond Breeze Unsweetened Original Almondmilk

- 1/3 cup almond butter

- 2 tablespoons rice wine vinegar

- 1 tablespoon soy sauce

- 1 teaspoon toasted sesame oil

- 1/2 teaspoon ground ginger

- (optional) 1 teaspoon sriracha

INSTRUCTIONS

TO MAKE THE SALAD:

1. Toss all ingredients together until evenly combined. Serve immediately.

TO MAKE THE CREAMY SESAME DRESSING:

1. Whisk all ingredients together until combined, adding in the sriracha if you would like a spicier dressing. Use immediately, or refrigerate in a sealed container for up to 1 day. (Also, if you

would like a sweeter dressing, feel free to stir in a few teaspoons of honey.)

MEDITERRANEAN FARRO SALAD

INGREDIENTS

SALAD INGREDIENTS:

- 3 cups chicken or vegetable stock

- 1 cup uncooked farro, rinsed and drained

- 1 large cucumber, seeded and finely-diced

- 2/3 cup finely-diced roasted red peppers

- 1/2 cup finely-diced sun-dried tomatoes

- 1/2 cup crumbled feta cheese

- half of a small red onion, finely diced (about 2/3 cup)

- 1/4 cup finely-chopped fresh parsley

- Greek vinaigrette (see ingredients below)

Greek Vinaigrette Ingredients:

- 3 Tablespoons olive oil

- 1 Tablespoon freshly-squeezed lemon juice

- 1 Tablespoon red wine vinegar

- 1/4 teaspoon dried oregano

- pinch of garlic powder

- pinch of salt

- pinch of black pepper

INSTRUCTIONS

TO MAKE THE SALAD:

1. Stir together stock and farro in a medium saucepan, and cook according to package instructions until al dente. Remove from heat, and drain off any extra stock once the farro is cooked. Let farro cool for at least 10 minutes.

2. Transfer farro to a large mixing bowl, and add in remaining ingredients, including the vinaigrette. Toss until combined.

3. Serve immediately, or cover and refrigerate for up to 2 days.

TO MAKE THE GREEK VINAIGRETTE:

1. Whisk all ingredients together until combined. Use immediately.

VEGGIE LOVERS' PASTA SALAD

INGREDIENTS

- 12 ounces dry pasta (I used farfalle)

- 2–3 tablespoons olive oil

- 1 zucchini, cut into bite-sized pieces

- 3 cups chopped broccoli florets (about 1 small head of broccoli)

- 2 bell peppers, cored and diced into bite-sized pieces (I used 1 yellow and 1 orange bell pepper)

- 1 cup cherry or grape tomatoes, halved

- 3 cloves garlic, peeled and minced

- salt and pepper

- half a small red onion, peeled and thinly-sliced

- 1/2 cup white balsamic vinaigrette (or any favorite balsamic or Italian dressing)

- optional topping: grated Parmesan cheese

INSTRUCTIONS

1. Cook the pasta in a large stockpot of generously-salted water al dente according to package directions. Drain pasta and rinse under cold water for about 20-30 seconds until no longer hot. Set aside.

2. Meanwhile, as your pasta water is heating and then your pasta is cooking, heat 1 tablespoon of oil in a large saute pan over medium-high heat. Add the zucchini and broccoli florets and saute for 3 minutes, stirring occasionally. Stir in the remaining oil, then add the bell peppers, tomatoes, garlic, and a few generous pinches of salt and pepper, and stir to combine. Continue sauteing for 4-5 more minutes, stirring occasionally, until the vegetables are cooked to your desired level of doneness. (I liked mine still slightly undercooked, so that they didn't get too

soft and mushy.) Stir in the red onion and saute for 1 more minute.

3. Then once the veggies and the pasta are all cooked, add them together in the large stockpot and drizzle with the vinaigrette. Toss until the pasta and veggies are evenly coated with the vinaigrette, and toss and then top with extra Parmesan if you'd like.

4. Serve immediately, or refrigerate in a sealed container for up to 3 days.

BLACK BEAN BURGERS

INGREDIENTS

- 1 tablespoon + 2 teaspoons olive oil, divided

- 4 ounces baby bella or white button mushrooms, finely chopped

- quarter of a small red onion, peeled and finely chopped (about 1/2 cup total)

- 2 cloves garlic, minced

- 1 (15-ounce) can black beans, rinsed and drained

- 2/3 cup Panko breadcrumbs*

- 1 egg white

- 2 teaspoons low-sodium steak seasoning (add more/less to taste)

- for serving: hamburger buns, Arla Muenster Sliced Cheese, fresh baby arugula, and/or other desired toppings

INSTRUCTIONS

1. Heat 2 teaspoons oil in a large saute pan over medium-high heat. Add mushrooms and onion and saute, stirring occasionally, for 4-5 minutes or until the onion is soft and translucent. Stir in garlic, and saute for 1-2 more minutes, stirring occasionally, until the garlic is fragrant. Remove mixture from heat, drain off any extra juices or oil, and set aside.

2. Meanwhile, as the mushroom mixture is cooking, add the black beans to a large mixing

bowl and roughly mash them with a potato masher (or the back of a spoon). Add in the cooked mushroom mixture, breadcrumbs, egg white, steak seasoning, and stir well until the mixture is evenly mixed. (If the mixture seems too wet, add in a few extra spoonfuls of breadcrumbs to help bind it together.)

3. Divide the mixture into four equal portions (each will be about 1/2 cup), and use your hands to form each portion into a large patty. Set aside.

4. Rinse out the saute pan, then return it to the stove and heat the remaining 1 tablespoon oil over medium-high heat. Carefully transfer the black bean burgers to the pan and cook on each side for 5-6 minutes, flipping once. If your pan is not big enough to fit all four burgers, you may need to do this in batches.

5. Remove from heat and serve the burgers on buns immediately, topped with Arla Muenster sliced cheese, fresh arugula, and/or any other toppings that sound good to you.

CHICKEN FLORENTINE GRILLED CHEESE

INGREDIENTS

- 2 teaspoons olive oil

- 1 small boneless skinless chicken breast*

- Kosher salt and freshly-cracked black pepper

- 2 slices of bread (I used sourdough)

- butter

- 3–4 Arla NaturallyGood Fontina Cheese Slices

- 2 tablespoons roughly-chopped sun-dried tomatoes

- 1 handful fresh baby spinach**

INSTRUCTIONS

1. Heat oil in a medium saute pan over medium-high heat. While the oil is heating, season the chicken with a generous pinch of salt and black pepper. Add the chicken to the pan and cook for 6-8 minutes, turning once, until the chicken is

cooked through and no longer pink on the inside. Remove pan from heat, then transfer the chicken to a cutting board and let it rest for 5 minutes. Then slice it into thin strips.

2. While the chicken is resting, butter one side of each piece of bread.

3. Place one slice (butter-side down) on your prep surface. Layer it evenly with 1-2 cheese slices, followed by the chicken slices, sun-dried tomatoes, spinach, and the remaining slice of bread (butter-side up).

4. Rinse out the saute pan (if needed), then return it to the stove over medium-high heat. Carefully transfer the sandwich to the pan and cook for 4-5 minutes on the first side, or until the bread is toasted and the cheese starts to melt. Carefully flip the sandwich to the other side, and cook for 3-4 minutes or until the bread is toasted.

5. Remove from pan, slice the sandwich down the middle, and serve warm.

SLOW COOKER APPLE CIDER PULLED PORK

INGREDIENTS

- 3.5 lb. pork shoulder

- 1 small white onion, thinly sliced

- 1 cup apple cider, homemade or store-bought

- 1/4 cup apple cider vinegar

- 1/4 cup brown sugar

- 2 tsp. ground cinnamon

- 2 tsp. kosher salt

- 1 tsp. black pepper

- 1 bay leaf

INSTRUCTIONS

1. Place half of the onions in the slow cooker. Set pork on top of onions, then cover pork with remaining onions.

2. In a separate bowl, whisk together all remaining ingredients. Pour on top of pork and onions.

3. Cook in the slow cooker on low for 6-8 hours, or until the pork is cooked and pulls apart easily with a fork. Shred pork using two forks, then toss once more in the juices so that it is coated. Serve warm.

4. You can also refrigerate or freeze the pork in a sealed container.

PORK AND BACON SLIDERS

INGREDIENTS

- 1 lb. ground pork

- salt and freshly-ground black pepper

- 2 Tbsp. vegetable or canola oil

- 6 slices of bacon, cooked and cut in half

- 10–12 slider buns or small rolls

- lettuce or spinach

- sliced tomatoes

- sliced cheddar cheese

- sliced white onions

INSTRUCTIONS

1. Season the ground pork with a few generous pinches of salt and freshly-ground black pepper. Score the mixture into 8 equal portions, and then use your hands to shape each portion into a patty.

2. Heat oil in a large skillet over medium-high heat. Cook the sliders in a single layer (you may need to do 2 or 3 batches) for about 3-4 minutes on each side, or until done to your taste. Once the sliders are done cooking, add the buns to the skillet (flat-side down) for a few seconds each until the insides are slightly brown and crispy.

3. Lay out the bottom halves of the buns on your work surface. Then add to each a layer of lettuce/spinach, onions, cheese, tomatoes, bacon, the pork patties, and then top with the

final layer of the bun. Secure with a toothpick and serve immediately.

PROSCIUTTO, PINEAPPLE & PESTO PANINIS

INGREDIENTS

• favorite sliced bread (I used sourdough)

• pesto, homemade or storebought

• fresh pineapple, cored and sliced into thick half-rings

• fresh mozzarella

• sliced prosciutto

INSTRUCTIONS

1. Spread a tablespoon or two of pesto on a slice of bread. Then layer on the pineapple, arranging to fit as needed. Then add a layer of mozzarella cheese, and then the sliced prosciutto. Repeat with additional paninis.

2. To make on a grill pan, heat the grill pan over medium-high heat. Add the paninis and cook until the bread is toasted. Remove and serve immediately.

3. To make in the oven, preheat the broiler to high. Add in the paninis and cook until the cheese is melted and the bread is toasted, about 2-4 minutes. (Keep a very close eye on these so that they do not burn!) Remove and serve immediately.

ROASTED BEET, ARUGULA, GOAT CHEESE & HONEY CROSTINI

INGREDIENTS

- 1 baguette or loaf of bread, sliced thin

- 4 medium-sized beets, peeled and diced (I used half red, half golden beets)

- 2 Tbsp. olive oil

- 4 oz. goat cheese (plain or herbed)

- 3 Tbsp. milk or cream

- 2 cups baby arugula

- honey, for drizzling

INSTRUCTIONS

1. Preheat oven to 425 degrees. Line a baking sheet with aluminum foil.

2. In separate mixing bowls (so that the colors do not bleed), toss each color of the diced beets with 1 Tbsp. olive oil. Spread each color of beets in an even layer on half of the baking sheet. Roast in the oven for 25-30 minutes, until tender when pierced with a fork. Remove and set aside.

3. Lower oven heat to 350. Then spread out bread slices in a single layer on a baking sheet, and bake for 10-15 minutes or until toasted. Remove and let cool.

4. Meanwhile, whisk together the goat cheese and milk in a small bowl until well-blended. Add more milk if you would like a thinner consistency for spreading.

5. Assemble the crostini by spreading a dollop of the goat cheese mixture on a piece of toasted bread, and then top with arugula and diced roasted beets. Drizzle with honey and serve.

BELL PEPPER EGG-IN-A-HOLE

INGREDIENTS

- 2 tsp. olive oil

- 1 bell pepper (any color), cut into four 1 cm-thick rings

- 4 large eggs

- coarse salt and ground pepper

- 1 Tbsp. grated Parmesan

- 4 slices multigrain bread, toasted

- 8 cups mixed salad greens

INSTRUCTIONS

1. In a large cast-iron or nonstick skillet, heat 1 teaspoon oil over medium-high heat. Add bell pepper, then crack 1 egg into the middle of each

pepper ring. Season with salt and pepper and cook until egg whites are mostly set but yolks are still runny, 2 to 3 minutes. Gently flip and cook 1 minute more for over easy.

2. Sprinkle with Parmesan and use a spatula to place each egg on a slice of toast. Toss salad greens with 1 teaspoon oil and season with salt and pepper; serve alongside eggs.

THAI CHICKEN QUESADILLAS

INGREDIENTS

- 2 tortillas (I used whole wheat)

- 2 Tbsp. peanut sauce, homemade or store-bought

- 1/4 cup cooked chicken, torn into bite-sized pieces

- 1 green onion, chopped

- half of a carrot, julienned (optional)

- small handful bean sprouts

- 1/2 cup mozzarella cheese, grated

- 2 Tbsp. peanuts

- 2 Tbsp. lightly packed fresh cilantro, stems removed

- 1 Tbsp. butter (optional)

INSTRUCTIONS

1. Lay out one tortilla on a flat working surface, and spread with the peanut sauce on top. Then sprinkle with the chicken, green onions, carrots, bean sprouts, mozzarella, peanuts and cilantro. Top with the remaining tortilla and gently press together.

2. Either in a skillet or grill pan, melt the butter and then add the quesadilla. Cook for about 2 minutes, and then carefully flip over and cook for another 2 minutes (or until tortilla begins to brown and cheese is melted).

3. OR, feel free to lay the quesadilla out on a cookie sheet, and bake in a 375 degree oven until the cheese is melted. (This is helpful for doing multiple quesadillas at a time!)

BRAID

INGREDIENTS

- 1 (13.8-ounce) can refrigerated pizza crust dough

- 1 Tbsp. olive oil

- 1/4 cup chopped onion

- 4 oz. spicy chicken sausage (or other sausage), chopped

- 2 large eggs, lightly beaten

- 1/2 cup (2 oz.) shredded Monterrey Jack cheese

- 1/2 cup shredded cheddar cheese

- 1/2 cup chopped seeded jalapeño peppers

- 1 large egg white, lightly beaten

INSTRUCTIONS

1. Preheat oven to 425°.

2. Unroll dough onto a baking sheet coated with cooking spray; pat into a 15 x 10-inch rectangle.

3. Heat oil in a large skillet over medium heat. Add onion and sausage; cook 9 minutes or until lightly browned. Stir in eggs; cook for 1 1/2 minutes or until set (while continuing to stir). Remove from heat.

4. Sprinkle Monterey Jack lengthwise down center of dough, leaving about a 2 1/2-inch border on each side. Spoon egg mixture evenly over cheese. Sprinkle cheddar over egg mixture; top with jalapeño peppers.

5. Make 2-inch-long diagonal cuts about 1 inch apart on both sides of dough to within 1/2 inch of filling using a sharp knife or kitchen shears. Arrange strips over filling, alternating strips diagonally over filling. Press ends under to seal. Brush with egg white. Bake at 425° for 15 minutes or until golden brown. Let stand 5 minutes. Cut crosswise into slices.

CHICKEN LETTUCE WRAPS

INGREDIENTS

CHICKEN STIR-FRY INGREDIENTS:

- 2 Tbsp. extra virgin olive oil

- 1 Tbsp. sesame oil

- 2 boneless skinless chicken breasts, cubed to 1/2?

- 1 (8 oz.) can sliced water chestnuts, drained and minced

- 1/2 cup mushrooms, minced

- 1/2 onion, chopped fine

- 3 cloves garlic, minced fine

- 6 large leaves of iceberg lettuce or nappa cabbage

STIR-FRY SAUCE INGREDIENTS:

- 1 Tbsp. soy sauce

- 1 Tbsp. brown sugar

- 1/2 teaspoon rice wine vinegar

POURING SAUCE INGREDIENTS:

- 1/4 cup sugar

- 1/2 cup warm water

- 2 Tbsp. tamari or soy sauce

- 2 Tbsp. rice wine vinegar

- 2 Tbsp. ketchup

- 1 Tbsp. lemon juice

- 1/4 tsp. sesame oil

- 1 Tbsp. Chinese or Dijon mustard (to taste – I'm not a big fan so only used 1 tsp.)

- 1 Tbsp. Sriracha (to taste – I used it all!)

- 2 cloves garlic, minced

INSTRUCTIONS

1. Begin by making the pouring sauce. In a large bowl, dissolve sugar in 1/2 cup warm water, then add soy sauce, rice wine vinegar, ketchup, lemon juice and sesame oil. Whisk together well. Then add in mustard and/or Sriracha to taste. Set aside or pop in the refrigerator until ready to use.

2. Combine olive oil and sesame oil and add to wok or large frying pan. Heat oil over high heat until it glistens, about one minute. Add chicken and saute until cooked through, then remove from the pan and cool. Keep oil in the pan, keeping it hot over a low flame.

3. Prep the stir fry sauce by mixing soy sauce, brown sugar, and rice vinegar in a small bowl.

4. Take pan that you cooked the chicken in (with the still-warming oil) and turn it up to medium-high heat. Add another tablespoon of olive oil to the pan, wait one minute, and then add garlic, onions, water chestnuts, mushrooms, and the stir-fry sauce you prepared earlier. Stir-fry everything until the mushrooms have cooked, about four minutes, then add in the chicken and stir until combined. Remove from heat.

5. Serve stir-fry with iceberg lettuce or nappa cabbage leaf wraps and top with pouring sauce.

PRESTO PESTO PANINI (WITH PROSCIUTTO, PROVOLONE & PEPPERS)

INGREDIENTS

- 1 ciabatta roll, individual-sized

- 2 slices prosciutto

- 1 slice provolone cheese

- 1–2 Tbsp. your favorite pesto sauce (classic basil pesto recipe)

- roasted red peppers (optional)

INSTRUCTIONS

1. Preheat panini grill (or grill pan, or George Foreman, or whatever you'd like to use!)

2. Slice ciabatta in half horizontally, and fill with layered prosciutto, provolone, pesto and red peppers. Fold together and grill for 5 minutes, or until bread is lightly golden and cheese is melted. Slice horizontally and serve.

SWEET PEA & RICOTTA CROSTINI

INGREDIENTS

- 1 baguette (sliced thin on a diagonal)

- 4 Tbsp. olive oil

- 1 (10 oz.) package frozen peas, thawed

- 1/2 cup ricotta (I used low-fat)

- 1 scallion (green onion), cut into 1" pieces

- 1 ounce Parmesan, cut into pieces (plus more grated Parmesan for topping)

- one squeeze of fresh lemon juice (optional)

- salt and pepper

INSTRUCTIONS

1. Heat oven to 375 degrees F. Place the baguette slices on a baking sheet and brush with 2 tablespoons of the oil. Toast until golden, about 10-12 minutes. (Watch carefully so they don't burn!)

2. Meanwhile, in a food processor fitted with the metal blade, puree the peas, ricotta, scallion, and Parmesan with the remaining 2 tablespoons of oil, lemon juice, salt (about 1/2 tsp.), and pepper (about 1/4 tsp.), scraping down the sides of the bowl occasionally, until the Parmesan is broken down and the mixture is nearly smooth.

3. Spread the pea mixture on the crostini and top with grated Parmesan, if desired.

WHOLE WHEAT PIZZA DOUGH

INGREDIENTS

- 1 cup warm* water

- 2 1/4 teaspoons (1 packet) active dry yeast

- 2 1/3 cups white whole wheat flour

- 2 tablespoons honey

- 1 tablespoon extra-virgin olive oil

- 1 1/2 teaspoons salt

- 3 tablespoons cornmeal

INSTRUCTIONS

1. Add warm water to the bowl of a stand mixer with the dough attachment, and sprinkle the yeast on top of the water. Give the yeast a quick stir to mix it in with the water. Then let it sit for 5-10 minute until the yeast is foamy.

2. Turn the mixer onto low speed, and add gradually flour, honey, olive oil and salt. Increase speed to medium-low, and continue mixing the dough for 5 minutes.

3. Remove dough from the mixing bowl, and use your hands to shape it into a ball. Grease the mixing bowl (or a separate bowl) with olive oil or cooking spray, then place the dough ball back in the bowl and cover it with a damp towel. Place in a warm location (I set mine by the window) and let it rise for 30-45 minutes until the dough has nearly doubled in size.

4. Preheat oven to 450 degrees F. Turn the dough onto a floured surface, and roll the dough into a 12- to 14-inch round for a thick-crusted pizza.

(Or cut the dough in half, and roll it into two 12-inch rounds for two thin crust pizzas.) Sprinkle a baking sheet or pizza stone evenly with the cornmeal, then place the dough on the baking sheet.

5. Top the dough with your desired sauce and toppings. (And for extra-golden crust, brush the crust with an extra few teaspoons of olive oil or butter.)

6. For thick crust, bake for 16-18 minutes, or until the crust is golden brown and the toppings are melted and cooked. For the (two) thin crusts, bake for 14-16 minutes, or until the crust is golden brown and the toppings are melted and cooked.

7. Slice and serve pizza warm.

BRUSSELS SPROUTS AND BACON FLATBREAD

INGREDIENTS

- 2 slices thick-cut bacon, diced

- 8 ounces Brussels Sprouts, thinly-sliced (with ends trimmed and discarded)

- 1 small red onion, peeled and thinly sliced

- 4 cloves garlic, peeled and thinly-sliced

- 2 pieces flatbread (I used store-bought naan)

- 1 tablespoon olive oil

- 1 cup shredded Mozzarella cheese

- 2 ounces crumbled goat cheese, blue cheese or feta cheese

- balsamic glaze*

INSTRUCTIONS

1. Preheat oven to 400°F.

2. Fry bacon in a large saute pan over medium-high heat until cooked. Transfer bacon to a separate plate with a slotted spoon, and set aside.

3. Meanwhile, keep about 1 tablespoon of the remaining bacon grease in the saute pan (you can discard the extra if there's too much grease in

there). Stir in the Brussels sprouts, red onion, and sliced garlic. Saute for 4-5 minutes, stirring frequently, until the mixture is softened and the garlic is fragrant. Remove from the heat and set aside.

4. Place the two pieces of flatbread on a large baking sheet, and brush the tops of each with olive oil. Sprinkle each piece of flatbread evenly with about 1/3 cup Mozzarella cheese, leaving a 1/2-inch border around the edges of the flatbread. Then divide the Brussels mixture, bacon and crumbled cheese evenly between the two pieces of flatbread, and spread them out evenly. Sprinkle with the remaining Mozzarella cheese.

5. Bake for 8-10 minutes, or until the Mozzarella has melted and the crusts are slightly golden.

6. Remove from the oven and drizzle with the balsamic glaze. Serve immediately.

www.ingramcontent.com/pod-product-compliance
Lightning Source LLC
Chambersburg PA
CBHW050824260726
48660CB00004B/1600